WELLNESS SIMPLIFIED

How Food affects

Moods, Bodies, and Behaviors

Suka Chapel-Horst, RN, PhD, QMHP, CPLT

WELLNESS SIMPLIFIED
How Food affects Moods, Bodies, and Behaviors

by Suka Chapel-Horst, RN, PhD, QMHP

Published by:
Brainworks Publishing
638 Spartanburg Highway, Suite #70-175
Hendersonville, NC 28792

WWW.IMRIWellness.org
www.BrainworksAlcoholRecovery.com

Neither the publisher nor the author is engaged in rendering professional advice or services to the individual reader. The ideas, procedures, and suggestions contained in this book are not intended as a substitute for consulting with your health care provider. All matters regarding your health require medical supervision. Neither the author nor the publisher shall be liable or responsible for any loss or damage allegedly arising from any information or suggestions in this book.

While the author has made every effort to provide accurate telephone numbers and Internet addresses at the time of publication, neither the publisher nor the author assumes any responsibility for errors, or for changes that occur after publication. Further, the publisher does not have any control over and does not assume any responsibility for author or third-party websites or their content.

ISBN-13 978-1495473760
ISBN-10 1495473767

ABOUT THE AUTHOR

As a child, one of my favorite stories was *The Little Engine That Could*. I still have that wonderful book. The little engine said, "I think I can; I think I can; I think I can". Today I'm saying, "Yes we can; yes we can; yes we can."

As a Registered Nurse and wellness educator for over forty five years, in the fields of mental health, criminal justice, and addictions, I've seen a major decline in the health of both adults and children. It hurts my heart to hear the stories of suffering and frustration.

The hurt is especially deep because most people are unaware of the cause of their suffering and so they fail to take the steps that can so easily and naturally free them from much of their pain and unhappiness.

My passion is to help people understand some of the underlying reasons for their physical, emotional, and mental pain and to help them begin the natural healing process leading to optimal health and wellness.

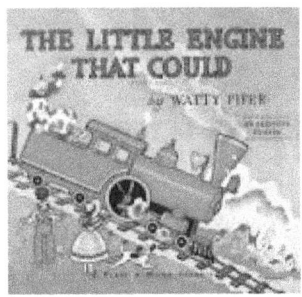

"Yes, we can."

Books and DVDs by Dr. Suka Chapel-Horst

WORKBOOKS
How to Quit Drinking for Good and Feel Good

"Why Do I Feel This Way?" Natural Healing for Optimal Health and Relief from Moods and Depression

BOOKS
Take a Leap of Faith

DVD

Depression – Ten Different Sources / Ten Different Approaches Your Guide to Finding and Treating the Real Underlying Cause

BOTTOM LINE BOOKS
BOOKS/DVD PowerPoint Presentations
Say Goodbye to Moods and Depression

PTSD – Alternative Resources for Recovery

The Real Cause and Solution for Alcohol Addiction

The Gift – A Sound Mind for Life

Cannabinoids: Marijuana, THC, CBN, Cannabis, CBD – The Hundredth Monkey Cure

Trick or Treat – What Your Doctor isn't Telling You about Mood Altering Medications

These books and DVD's can be ordered through:
www.IMRIWellness.org
www.AriseAlcoholRecovery.com or by calling 417-380-3254

ACKNOWLEDGEMENTS

I want to thank all the pioneers in the fields of wellness, nutritional health, and Integrative Medicine who have dedicated their lives to research and teaching so that we can have a deeper understanding of the underlying cause of illness, disease, and mental disorders. In particular, I am grateful for the support, mentoring, and friendship of Barbara Reed Stitt, PhD, one of the early messengers of the power of foods to affect behavior. Her book *Food & Behavior* is a classic. Most importantly, I am ever grateful and appreciative for the never-failing support from David, my husband, best friend, and partner, who shares my passion for teaching and healing.

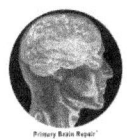

PRIMARY BRAIN REPAIR

Primary Brain Repair focuses on providing the brain, body, and spirit with the basic requirements for health and wellbeing. It's the first line response to all illnesses and disorders. It involves the use of natural micronutrients, nutrition therapy, exercise, and stress relief.

Optimal health can be achieved by most people by following these guidelines. For individuals who need more intensive treatment, these basic health steps will be the foundation that allows advanced treatment to be effective. When primary brain repair is not addressed, medications and counseling have little long-term effect.

Using simple, but effective, recovery tools, *Primary Brain Repair* will improve the health of everyone who applies it. How can that be? Simply, because we go back to the basics of how the brain and body are designed to work. The answer is in nature, and the method is natural.

At Integrative Memory Research Institute our mission and passion is to educate the public and healthcare professionals about the most advanced methods for obtaining optimal health, naturally. Based on the latest neuroscience and biochemical research, along with years of experience, Dr. Suka offers leading-edge knowledge and how-to information to those who are seeking real recovery versus symptom relief.

We are passionate about helping you. That's why we've created self-help books and DVDs to guide you through the process.

www.IMRIWellness.org
417-380-3254

INTRODUCTION

We are a nation of "sick puppies". I'm referring to the rapidly increasing numbers of children and adults suffering from illness, disease, mental misery, and premature aging, but the cause isn't a secret and the cure isn't rocket science.

It all starts in the home with what we're eating and what we're teaching our children about health and wellness. Optimal health can almost be as simple as "Chicken soup and an apple a day".

What we need to understand is that our unhealthy moods, bodies, and behaviors are often the result of what we're eating, or not eating. For example, a child's tantrum can be due to an overdose of sugar from fruit juice. Asthma can be the reaction to a wheat allergy, and anger and aggression can be due to heavy milk drinking. Oops! What's that?

Yes, we are what we eat, physically, emotionally, and mentally. Before seeking medications to treat symptoms, we can usually relieve the symptoms naturally by eating nutritious foods. Our bodies aren't made of Prozac. They're made of healthy foods and nutrients. How simple is that?

"Dr. Suka" Chapel-Horst
February 2014
Etowah, North Carolina

WELLNESS SIMPLIFIED

How Food affects
Moods, Bodies, and Behaviors

Let's begin with some current trends. The U.S. is 1st in healthcare spending but is 37th in world health. World Health Organization, 2000 And, despite the high cost of healthcare, Americans have increasing levels of illness, disease, mental misery, and premature aging. Just consider some of these statistics.

35.8% of Americans are obese and 68% are overweight. (Obesity means 20% over normal weight or 30 pounds overweight, depending on sex, height, build, and age.) The U.S. is the most malnourished country in the world.

Up to 80% of Americans admit to having some level of the blues, blahs, moodiness or chronic depression. 46.7 million antidepressant prescriptions were sold in 2011, a 9.1% rise over 2010.

Recent Mayo Clinic research indicates that 70% of Americans are taking one prescription drug, 50% are taking two prescription drugs, and 20% of Americans are taking five or more prescription drugs. CBS News 6/20/2013

What about our children?
- 11% have ADD/ADHD
- 1 in 88 have Autism or Asperger's Disorder
- 8.3% have Type 1 Diabetes
- 18% have an Anxiety Disorder
- 10.2% have an Oppositional Defiant Disorder

In 2010 an estimated 22.1 million persons had a substance addiction or substance abuse problem. That's 8.7 percent of the population aged 12 or older. Of that number, 17.9 million Americans are addicted to alcohol. *Diagnostic and Statistical Manual of Mental Disorders*, 4th Edition, DSM-IV

Projections by the U.S. Government Center for Disease Control are that:
- Obesity will increase from 36% to 42% by 2030
- Diabetes will increase from 8.3% to 33% by 2050
- Cancer will increase from 25% to 45% by 2030
- Alzheimer's will increase from 5.4 million to 10.8 million by 2030

Can we change these figures and halt this terrible progression of worsening health? The answer is *"Yes, we can"*.

Dr. Barbara Reed Stitt, a pioneer in the field of food and behavior, has been a major force for positive change in criminal justice and school system approaches to nutrition and behavior. Her classic book, *Food & Behavior,* gained international recognition.

Dr. Stitt begins her book with this story. Twenty-three year old Raymond (not his real name), in a jealous rage with his girlfriend, pulled out a gun, pointed it at her head and intentionally pulled the trigger. She deflected the gun but the bullet tore a one-inch hole in her left hand. Ruth, the girlfriend (not her real name), refused to press charges so Raymond was delivered to Dr. Stitt, who was the Chief Probation Officer in the Cuyahoga Falls, Ohio, Municipal Court.

In their first conversation Dr. Stitt noticed that Raymond was detached, anxious, and mentally confused. He admitted to having uncontrollable emotions, violent anger, and suicidal thoughts. He also had severe abdominal pain.

When Dr. Stitt asked him what he usually ate, he reported that he lived on donuts, pastry, white bread, pasta, processed canned goods, candy, and gallons of coffee. Just before the shooting, Raymond and his girlfriend had eaten fast food. Later tests showed that he also had excessive toxins in his body due, in part, to his heavy inhalation of gunpowder fumes when he practiced marksmanship.

Instead of sending him to counseling, Dr. Stitt put Raymond on a healthy nutritional and food supplement plan which included eating three meals a day, plus healthy snacks in between his meals. He followed the plan and became a healthy, productive member of society with no further criminal behaviors. To his amazement, Raymond's entire personality and quality of life changed for the better. (The book *Food & Behavior* is available at BrainworksRecovery.com)

WE ARE WHAT WE EAT

Most Americans are addicted to sugar. **Sugar** is the number one destroyer and it's four times more addictive than cocaine. Excess sugar is a drug that is responsible for mood swings and personality changes, sometimes going from nice to nasty in a moment. Something as simple as eating lots of candy or heavy milk drinking can lead to domestic violence and criminal behavior.

Before 1890 we consumed approximately 20 pounds of sugar a year. Today people consume an average of 135 pounds of sugar yearly. Many criminals are eating as much as 300 pounds of sugar a year, a major contributor to their criminal behavior.

Some of the results of this huge intake of sugar are:

- Obesity
- Asthma
- Arthritis
- Diabetes
- Gall stones
- Cancer
- Hypertension
- Heart disease
- Dementia
- Alzheimer's

HYPOGLYCEMIA

Approximately 80% of Americans are hypoglycemic meaning that they have low blood sugar. The pancreas releases insulin in order to digest the sugar we eat. When a lot of sugar is being consumed on a regular basis, there is an overproduction of insulin which cries out for more sugar. When a person has low blood sugar they can experience:

- Cravings
- Depression
- Constant worrying
- Unprovoked anxieties
- Exhaustion
- Mental confusion
- Forgetfulness
- Irritability
- Insomnia
- Internal trembling

When normal glucose, or blood sugar, levels are flooding the entire brain, people have the mental ability to be socially responsible. But when there is low blood sugar, it will go to a more primitive part of the brain whose sole function is survival. They will then be in survival mode with fight or flight, gut reactions and these can include anger and violence. Road rage, domestic abuse, manslaughter, and unintended suicide are examples of the actions of

14

people who are in a severely hypoglycemic state, as Raymond was when he attempted to kill his girlfriend.

People with no intention or plans to suicide have taken their lives while in a severe hypoglycemic state because of deep depression that overwhelms them. They have so little blood sugar in the thinking part of the brain that they can't weigh the consequences of their actions or see the future in a more balanced way. This is a major cause of unplanned teenage suicides. It's very sad and so very preventable when we understand that the cause is related to junk foods, fast foods, too much soda, and just too much sugar in all its forms.

For example, the sugar in Coca Cola:
- 12 oz. bottle has 140 Calories from sugar or 2 Tablespoons
- 20 oz. bottle has 240 Calories from sugar or 1/3 cup
- 1 Liter bottle has 400 Calories from sugar or 1/2 cup

The sugar in Mountain Dew:
- 12 oz. bottle has 170 Calories from sugar or 1/4 cup
- 20 oz. bottle has 290 Calories from sugar or > 1/3 cup
- 34 oz. bottle has 440 Calories from sugar or < 2/3 cup

There is 40% more caffeine and 15% more sugar in Mountain Dew than there is in a Coke. How many people are drinking one or more liters of cola every day? Their moods, bodies, and behaviors, and lives are being negatively affected by all that sugar.

Little children are being fed apple juice by moms who think it's good for them but are unaware that there is approximately one tablespoon of sugar in every eight ounces of juice. Many children become addicted to sugar before the age of two and we see the effects in tantrums, poor grades, aggressive behaviors, and early addictions to alcohol and other drugs.

Food manufacturers attempt to hide the fact that processed food is highly, if not, mostly, sugar. Just look at the growing list of sugar names.

LIST OF JUST SOME SUGAR NAMES

Agave nectar	Demerara Sugar	Golden sugar	Molasses
Barbados Sugar	Dextrin	Golden syrup	Muscovado sugar
Barley malt	Dextran	Granulated sugar	Organic raw sugar
Beet sugar	Dextrose	Grape sugar	Panocha
Blackstrap Molasses	Diastatic malt	Grape juice	Powdered sugar
Brown sugar	Diatase	concentrate	Raw sugar
Buttered syrup	D-mannose	HFCS	Refiner's syrup
Cane crystals	Evaporated cane juice	High-Fructose	Rice Syrup
Cane juice crystals	Ethyl maltol	Corn Syrup	Sorbitol
Cane sugar	Florida Chrystals	Honey	Sorghum syrup
Caramel	Free Flowing	Icing sugar	Splenda
Carob syrup	Fructose	Invert sugar	Sucrose
Castor sugar	Fruit juice	Lactose	Sugar
Confectioner's sugar	Fruit juice	Malt syrup	Syrup
Corn syrup	concentrate	Maltodextrin	Table sugar
Corn sweetener	Galactose	Maltose	Treacle
Corn syrup solids	Glucose	Mannitol	Turbinado sugar
Crystalline fructose	Glucose solids	Artificial Maple	Yellow sugar
Date sugar		Syrup	

INGREDIENTS: MILLED CORN, SUGAR, CORN SYRUP, MOLASSES, SALT, PARTIALLY HYDRO-GENATED VEGETABLE OIL (ONE OR MORE OF: COCONUT, COTTONSEED, AND SOYBEAN)***, SODIUM ASCORBATE AND ASCORBIC ACID (VITAMIN C), NIACINAMIDE, ZINC OXIDE, REDUCED IRON, WHEAT STARCH, PYRIDOXINE HYDROCHLO-RIDE (VITAMIN B6), RIBOFLAVIN (VITAMIN B2), THIAMIN HYDROCHLORIDE (VITAMIN B1), VITAMIN A PALMITATE, BHT (PRESERVATIVE), ANNATTO COLOR, FOLIC ACID, VITAMIN D AND VITAMIN B12.
*** ADDS A NEGLIGIBLE AMOUNT OF FAT.
†LESS THAN 0.5g TRANS FAT PER SERVING

This food label shows that the first four ingredients in this product are sugar (corn is sugar). Whatever this product is, it's really an addictive drug that can change one's reactions and behaviors, without warning.

If children are having tantrums, acting out, bullying, feeling depressed or are overly sensitive, check out what they are eating. Sugar may very well be one of the reasons for their behavior.

Sugar is in all white foods such as ice cream, pasta, white bread, pizza crust, white rice, white potatoes, and white flour baked goods. To reach optimal health, we have to cut way down or quit eating these non-foods. After you've weaned yourself off them, you won't miss them. Really! Once optimal health is gained, it won't hurt to have some fast food on a rare occasion, but you won't crave it and you may not even like it anymore.

In the 1990's I founded and directed a wellness program in five centers in Minneapolis and St. Paul, MN called *PEERS Optimal Health Program*. (PEERS meant "We are all equals, or peers, in this program".)

One of the participants was Sue Ricker, (name given with her permission) who had lived with a severe case of Candida for months. Candida, a very common yeast overgrowth in the intestine, is fed by sugar. It causes a whole host of nasty and painful emotional, mental, and physical problems. (See the book "Why Do I Feel This Way?" for a list of symptoms and a self-test.)

Sue had been unable to find relief until she began this program. After a few weeks on the program she wrote me, *"I am constantly amazed how such a simple change in diet can have such a drastic, yet wonderful impact on everything I feel and do."*

The changes Sue experienced, in her own words, were:

- More alert
- More creative
- Clearer thinking
- Better memory
- More energy
- More active
- Sleep better
- Less stressed
- React more calmly
- Migraines seldom
- Less bloated
- Less gassy
- Eat less
- Weight melts off
- Gone plugged ears
- Rare sinus congestion
- Clearer skin
- Eyes stay open
- Normalized periods
- PMS symptoms reduced

"When I choose to eat 'forbidden foods', the results are a shocking reminder of why I take the extra time to stay healthy. I am so happy to be me again," wrote Sue.

Recently, my own doctor, an internist, said, "If everyone cut down on sugar, I'd lose 70% of my patients." Is that a telling statement? Quite possibly, sugar may be our number one enemy, even affecting how politicians and government officials perform their work. Hmm.

The **Standard American Diet**, or **SAD**, appropriately named, consists of low-grade burgers, chicken nuggets, processed cheese, white bread, fries, and cola for starters. Whole families live almost entirely on fast food and junk food. Chips, candy, cookies, doughnuts, jugs of coffee, and jumbo sized bottles of cola are standard fare in many homes, which is why America is the most malnourished country in the world, and why we have a high infant mortality rate, along with climbing rates of ADD/ADHD, diabetes, obesity, cancer, heart disease, and Alzheimer's. This junk food diet is also responsible, in part, to the increasing rate of violence in America.

Appetite stimulants are chemicals that are added to foods to make us feel hungry, even when our bodies don't need more food. One of the reasons why we have such a high obesity rate is that fast food chains and food manufacturers include these appetite stimulants in their foods so that people will eat more.

Appetite stimulants are in almost all processed foods including Oreo Cookies, potato chips, snacks, ice cream, pizza, lunch meats, packaged foods and more. The result is that people eat too much. It's hard to eat just one potato chip, isn't it?

Non-foods include white foods, processed foods, chemicals, preservatives, food coloring, fake food, some cooking oils, and hydrogenated foods such as margarine. Avoid dinner mixes, processed cheese and processed lunch meat including most hot dogs. (There are hot dogs that are free of chemicals and preservatives.) Also avoid highly sugared and colored cereals. Think those blueberries in cereal and muffin mixes are good for you? Surprise. They aren't blueberries. They're made of compacted grain and are filled with toxic food coloring.

> *Constant consumption of sugar, fast food, and junk food leads to fast reactions and junk behaviors.*

GMO's, or genetically modified organisms, are plants or animals that have been genetically engineered with DNA from bacteria, viruses or other plants and animals. GMO's are designed to withstand the direct application of an herbicide, and/or to produce an insecticide. More than sixty countries around the world have banned GMO's but the FDA allows GMO foods in the U.S. There is a movement in our country to have GMO products labeled but so far, most are not.

When insects eat genetically modified crops, the insect's bellies explode. Shortly before slaughtering, cows are fed GMO corn to fatten them up, but the cows must be killed in a timely fashion to avoid becoming sick, and therefore, unsalable. When we eat corn-fed cattle, the genes are passed on to us.

When humans eat genetically modified food, or meat from cattle which have been fed the GMO's, they are ingesting the modified gene, as well. As with the insects and cattle, the modified genes enter human intestines with the result that normal, healthy bacteria in human intestines are destroyed. This creates intestinal problems in humans, leading to a whole host of physical disorders.

GMO linked disorders include:
- Allergies
- Asthma
- Autism
- Cancer
- Infertility
- Decreased immunity
- Leaky gut
- Organ damage
- Spontaneous abortions
- Tissue damage
- BEHAVIORAL DISORDERS

Another problem is GMO's effect on human fertility. For example, in a controlled study, the first offspring of mice which had been fed GMO's were born smaller than control groups without GMO's. The third generation of mice were infertile. naturalfertilityinfo.com

GMO foods to avoid are:

- Soy (Soy in infant milk is the source of many problems.)
- Corn
- High fructose corn syrup/corn sugar
- Cottonseed
- Canola oil   (derived from Rapeseed)
- Sugar beets (Most sugar in foods come from sugar beets.)
- Potatoes
- Hawaiian papaya
- Zucchini (some)
- Squash (some)
- Salmon (some)
- Beef
- Milk (BGH – Bovine Growth Hormone)
- Dairy (BGH – Bovine Growth Hormone)

Reactions to **Food Coloring** are the same as allergic reactions to foods. Food coloring is found in:

- Candy
- Cereals
- Crackers
- Breads
- Cheeses
- Popsicles
- Ice creams
- Processed foods
- Food supplements (Some children's vitamins, for example)
- Over-the-counter drugs (Cough syrups, etc.)
- ...and many more

MSG or Monosodium Glutamate is a flavor enhancer frequently used in Asian foods. Common reactions are:

- Headache
- Flushing
- Sweating
- Chest pain
- Nausea
- Weakness
- Joint Pain
- Rashes
- Rapid heartbeat

MSG isn't limited to Asian foods. It's also found in all of the following:

- Corn starch
- Corn syrup
- Modified food starch
- Dextrose
- Rice syrup
- Brown rice syrup
- Milk powder
- Reduced fat milk (skim, 1%, and 2% fat milk)
- Most things "low fat" or "no fat"
- Anything "enriched"
- Anything "vitamin enriched"
- Anything "pasteurized"
- Annatto (food coloring)
- Vinegar& Balsamic vinegar

And finally, **Toxic Substances** can be devastating, as well. They include:

- Molds
- Chemicals such as fluoride in city water systems
- Heavy metals including lead
- Mercury in dental fillings
- Pesticides
- Herbicides

Infra-Red, Dry-Heat Saunas, frequently found at local YMCA's, are an enjoyable and excellent way to release toxins and reduce stress.

FOOD AND WELLNESS – THE SOLUTION

We begin our wellness program by eating three wholesome meals every day beginning with breakfast, the most important meal of the day. Just think, if our last meal was in the early evening and it's now 8 am, we may have gone up to twelve hours without food. We are hypoglycemic in the morning, due to low blood sugar. If we wait another four or five hours before eating, we may drink too much caffeine or grab something sweet. You already know what low blood sugar can do to a person.

To prevent this, eat a healthy breakfast that includes both protein and healthy fat. Protein and fat take longer to digest than other foods, so they keep us from craving sweets. Failure to eat a healthy breakfast is a major reason why people with addictions relapse. Failure to eat breakfast leads to weight gain, obesity, and diabetes due to the effects of chronic hypoglycemia.

That **caffeine** drink some people "have to have" in the morning releases stored emergency sugar into the brain, providing a temporary lift. But it also creates more cravings for sweets to replace the emergency sugar that was used up. Too many people think a good breakfast consists of "coffee and doughnuts". One might as well be taking a snort of cocaine, for all the good it's doing for the brain and body. Coffee and doughnuts are drugs that are causing emotional, mental, and physical misery over time. If you love coffee, stick to just one or two cups of it, along with a healthy breakfast including protein and natural fat, such as eggs and butter.

> *A healthy diet consists of protein,*
> *natural fats, vegetables, fruits, and grains.*

Protein is life. Protein is in every living cell. A stone has no protein and so it isn't a living substance. Without adequate protein, we die. If we are low in protein, we can experience these symptoms:

- Anxiety
- Irritability
- Depression
- Poor concentration
- Low energy
- Low motivation
- Put on weight easily
- Impatience
- Impulsiveness
- Cravings sweets
- Insomnia (This is the most unreported symptom in the U.S.)
- Overwhelmed
- Frustrated
- Persistent emotional pain
- Persistent physical pain

Healthy sources of protein are:
- Nuts
- Beans
- Butter (100% natural)
- Cheese (Avoid processed cheeses)
- Yogurt   (Buy organic, low-sugar products without fruit.)
- Non-Denatured Whey powder (Not usually found in stores)
- Fish
- Turkey
- Free range chicken and eggs
- Beef from grass fed cows   (Avoid all processed lunch meats.)

Healthy fats are a must for wellness. Our brain is about 60% fat and our brain cells require healthy fat to operate efficiently. Years ago we were misled into thinking that fat was dangerous for our hearts and blood vessels, so we bought the false notion that hydrogenated fats were better for us than natural fats. In fact, since the advent of hydrogenated margarine and saturated oils, heart disease and strokes have increased, not decreased. Dr. Atkins was right, and ahead of his time.

Healthy fats include:
- 100% fat butter (if not allergic)
- Almond milk
- Olives
- Avocados
- Eggs from free range, organically fed chickens.
- Peanut and other nut butters (if not allergic)
- Cheese (if not allergic) Avoid all processed cheeses.
- Chicken fat and chicken soup

When cooking, use real butter or coconut oil. Olive oil and vinegar are excellent for salad dressings but even olive oil is unhealthy when heated. Avoid all hydrogenated fats and all oils derived from corn or cottonseed.

> *A diet rich in healthy fats, veggies and fruit reduces the chance of dementia by 44%, according to a recent Mayo Clinic report.*

Eat **FRESH vegetables and fruits,** organic when possible. The best sources are local farmer's markets. To avoid ingesting harmful pesticides, herbicides, and bacteria, wash all produce under water for 30 seconds before peeling or eating.

Avoid canned fruits as they tend to have a high sugar content. Vegetables used to be canned in glass. The coating used to preserve metal cans from corroding is highly toxic to some people. Canned vegetables, while convenient to store, should be a last choice for healthy nutrition. Check labels for sodium content and choose low-sodium products when available.

Healthy snacks between meals include:
- Nuts
- Cheese
- Hard boiled eggs
- Chicken (not nuggets!!!)
- Yogurt (Without fruit)
- Peanut butter (if not allergic)
- Almond and other nut butters (if not allergic)
- Carrots with nut butter
- Celery with nut butter

Beryl Westphal, RN, ANP, is a Neurology Nurse Practitioner (name given with permission) who was a participant in my PEERS Optimal Health Program in Minneapolis. When she first came to the program her symptoms included:

- Severe abdominal pain
- Overweight
- Left arm, neck, and shoulder pain

Beryl stopped drinking caffeine, took a generous amount of suggested supplements, followed a healthy nutritional program, and exercised.

The results she experienced in nine months were:

- No abdominal or intestinal discomfort
- No sugar cravings
- 33 pound weight loss
- 80% pain reduction in her neck and shoulder

Beryl's weight loss was slow and steady, helping to assure that she wouldn't regain it. It reflected a healthy diet, not a gimmick diet leading to rapid weight gain, frustration, disappointment, and further loss of self-esteem.

Beryl understood that the muscle pain she was experiencing was due to stress. She was using stress reduction exercises, along with massage, and was continuing to notice a decreasing level of frustration and stress in her life as time went on.

Malnutrition affects perhaps 80% of Americans. Proof of that is in the large increase in the number of doctor visits and hospital admissions. Obesity, a sign of malnutrition, is projected to reach 42% of Americans by 2030.

Who's at fault? There are many causes, and most are not due to the fault of individuals. I lay the majority of blame on a lack of education from schools and the medical profession, that are themselves ignorant of the cause of much of the physical, emotional, and mental disorders so many are suffering from.

As long as the agricultural and pharmaceutical industries have a tight grip on food, medicine and politicians, we will have to get smart on our own and refuse to become the "sheeple" they want us to be.

Farms aren't what they used to be. Crops no longer have healthy nutrients due to failure to rotate crops, failure to allow land to remain fallow every few years, and the intense use of insecticides, herbicides, and other growth chemicals, not to mention acid rain and poor water quality. The only healthy answer is to "eat organic" and to supplement our diet with neuronutrients, or brain food.

Is there such a thing as a magic bullet? Of course not, however, food supplements come as close to being magic bullets, as we can get.

Food Supplements are the amino acids, vitamins, minerals, enzymes, essential fatty acids, and trace elements that our bodies are made of. Babies are not made from Prozac. They're made from the food the mother eats. If that food can build the wondrous creation of a living being, why do we switch to synthetic molecules (medicines) for maintaining good health after birth?

Even animal food has nutrients added, as much as 30% according to some products. Are our pets eating better than we are? Perhaps so.

Just how important are these nutrients? Well, let's look at just the **Vitamin B's.** When there is a deficiency in these nutrients, multiple symptoms may develop such as:

Emotional Symptoms due to a Vitamin B Deficiency:
- Confusion
- Poor concentration
- Poor memory
- Depression
- Insomnia
- Anxiety
- Agitation
- Impulsiveness
- Anger
- Irritability
- Quarrelsome
- Mood swings
- Panic attacks
- Obsessive-compulsiveness

Physical Symptoms due to a Vitamin B Deficiency
- Hyperactivity
- Headache
- Fatigue
- Insomnia
- Convulsions
- Decreased sex drive
- Tension
- Dizziness
- Gastric ulcers

- High blood pressure
- High cholesterol
- Arteriosclerosis
- Constipation
- Hair loss
- Skin eruptions
- Kidney /Liver impairment
- Extreme nervous exhaustion

How many times does a person go to the doctor complaining about some of these symptoms and the doctor just hands out a prescription to halt the symptom, when the real cause is simply a lack of Vitamin B's?

> *The first question every doctor ought to ask is,*
> *"What are you eating?"*

What happens when we aren't getting enough protein, or the amino acids which make up the protein?

Symptoms of Amino Acid Deficiencies (Low Protein)
- Anxiety
- High stress
- Tension
- Depression
- Fatigue
- Insomnia
- Tremors
- Irritability
- Sudden anger
- Violent outbursts

- High distractibility
- Poor concentration
- Short-term memory loss

Did you know that:
1. **Alcohol** flushes proteins and Vitamin B's out of the body.
2. **Sugar** removes Vitamin B's, calcium, and magnesium from the body and...
3. **Caffeine** depletes the body of:
   - Vitamin B's
   - Vitamin C
   - Magnesium
   - Zinc
   - Calcium
   - Potassium and...
   - Caffeine also leads to hypoglycemia, or low blood sugar.

Vitamin D, which comes from the sun, is very important for our overall health but few of us in the northern hemisphere get enough of it, especially in the winter, which is why some people have winter blues or Seasonal Affective Disorder, even if they live in Florida.

To learn more about Vitamin D, go to www.vitamindcouncil.org. You can get Vitamin D testing through them, as well. Vitamin D is so important that I've devoted a whole chapter to it in my book *"Why Do I Feel This Way?" – Natural Healing for Optimal Health and Relief from Moods and Depression.* (See Resources.)

A Vitamin D Deficiency leads to:

- Arthritis
- Alzheimer's
- Rheumatoid arthritis
- Autoimmune diseases
- Cancers
- Depression
- Diabetes
- Emphysema
- Chronic bronchitis
- Fibromyalgia
- Gout
- Kidney disease
- Lupus
- Parkinson's
- PMS
- Fetal developmental deficiencies
- Schizophrenia development later in life is increased if the pregnant mother is Vitamin D deficient
- Tuberculosis
- **Seasonal Affective Disorder (SAD)**

So, what's the solution? In order to be fully healthy, alert, and alive, we must add nutritional food supplements to our diet. I've put together a list of the most **BASIC** nutrients necessary for optimal health. Most health-conscious people add several more supplements to their diet but for starters, this list can make a big difference in how you feel, physically, emotionally and mentally.

Basic Supplements for Adults

- Vitamin B6 150 mg daily

- Vitamin B12 1000 mcg daily

- Vitamin C 1000 mg twice daily, preferably sustained release to get a longer-lasting effect. (If diarrhea occurs, decrease the dosage until it is gone.)

- Vitamin D3   5000 IU – 20,000 IU daily.
  (We can take up to 40,000 IU daily for several months without any negative effects.)

  If you are experiencing any of the symptoms or disorders I listed for Vitamin D deficiency, start taking 20,000 IU daily for four or more weeks and notice how you feel. As your symptoms decrease you can ease back down to 5000 IU and use that as your maintenance dose, increasing it as needed. There are no negative side effects from Vitamin D.

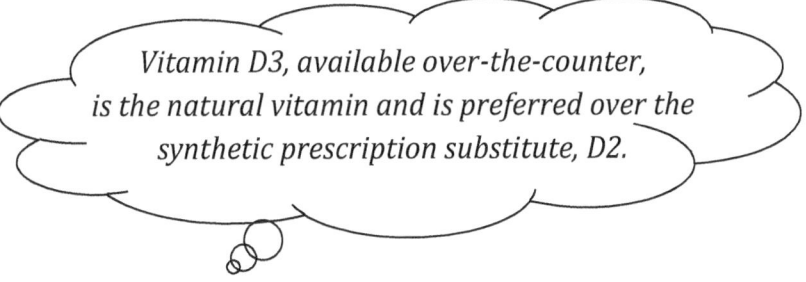

Vitamin D3, available over-the-counter, is the natural vitamin and is preferred over the synthetic prescription substitute, D2.

- OMEGA 3 with DHA 1000 mg twice daily

- Multi Vitamin daily (good quality)

Basic Supplements for Children Above Age One

- Vitamin B Complex   1 daily

- Vitamin C 1000 mg twice daily, preferably sustained release to get a longer-lasting effect. (If diarrhea occurs, decrease the dosage until it is gone.)

- Vitamin D3   Up to 2,000 IU during first year of age is safe. For children age 1 to 12 years, 5,000 IU of Vitamin D3 a day is safe. Michael F. Holic, PhD, MD, a pioneer of vitamin d research, Life Extension Magazine, September 2010.

  Teenagers and adults need a total of at least 5,000 IU of Vitamin D3 a day. All teenagers and adults can easily tolerate 20,000 IU of Vitamin D3 a day without concern for toxicity. An optimal blood level of 25-hydroxyvitamin D3 is 80- 100 ng/ml in teenagers and adults. Paul Stitt, PhD, Pioneer in Vitamin D research

- Multi Vitamin daily (good quality)

Charlee Carlson, another of the participants in my PEERS program (name given with permission), used an inhaler for severe asthma and wheezing. At my suggestion, she started using cayenne pepper, a NATURAL food supplement. In five days her doctor could find no signs of bronchial spasms or mucus. Her asthma symptoms were completely gone. This is another example of the value of natural food supplements.

> *When purchasing food supplements,*
> *always choose quality over cost.*

The cheapest supplements are made in China. There is no quality control, no supervision, and no oversight in the manufacturing process. Upon inspection, many of these supplements have been found to have none of the ingredients listed on the packaging! Shop wisely, not cheaply.

Allergies, alone, can be responsible for almost any and all symptoms. Any food can be an allergen.

The **Eight Most Common Food Allergens Are:**

- Dairy
- Wheat
- Eggs
- Peanuts
- Tree nuts
- Soy
- Fish
- Shell fish

An ever increasing number of adults and children are allergic to foods, but many aren't aware that it's the foods they're eating that are the source of their symptoms. Perhaps one of the most severe allergies is from dairy products.

Dairy Allergy Symptoms (Think especially about children)

- Hyperactivity
- Lack of attention (Think poor school grades)
- Lack of impulse control
- Mood swings
- Violence/Aggression (Think bullying)
- Headaches
- Sleep problems

In her book, *Food & Behavior*, Dr. Barbara Reed Stitt cites statistics that prison inmates drink twice as much milk as the normal population and that their allergies to milk often lead to violent and aggressive behaviors. Experiments have shown that when milk is withdrawn from their diet, prison violence decreases.

Unless **Breads** and **Cereals** are made from sprouted grains, the following chain-reactions created by too much grain consumption are shown to increase the risk of:

- Anxiety
- Diabetes
- Depression
- Autism
- Allergies
- Infertility
- Obesity
- Arthritis
- Schizophrenia (100% are allergic to gluten. Once off gluten, some individuals become completely symptom free.)
- Autoimmune diseases
- Various cancers including pancreatic, colon, stomach and lymphoma

Hospital admissions have increased seven fold in the last decade due to severe allergic reactions.

When people are allergic to a food, they eat a lot of that food on a regular basis. They crave that food and don't want to give it up. The reason is that when they go without the food, they experience detoxifying symptoms that are often very uncomfortable. If they immediately restart the offending food, those detoxifying symptoms disappear. However, the ongoing allergic reactions continue or become worse the longer a person remains on the offending foods.

As people withdraw and detoxify from foods to which they are allergic, any number of mild to severe symptoms can occur. However, as soon as the detoxifying state is over, usually in two to four days, they begin to feel better and their ongoing symptoms begin to diminish. If they once again eat the offending food, the negative allergic reactions return and that's how they know they are allergic to a food.

Allergic Symptoms can include:
- Attention deficit
- Chronic fatigue syndrome
- Depression
- Migraines
- Hyperactivity
- Insomnia
- Learning disorders
- Irritability
- Angry outbursts
- Asthma
- Constipation
- Diarrhea
- Low energy
- Angry
- Joint pain
- Poor concentration
- Cravings

From 1997 to 2011 food allergies in children increased by 50% due to the increased consumption of sodas, junk and fast foods, sugar, food coloring, additives, and GMO foods and grains.

Behavioral Symptoms of Children with Allergies

From *THE IMPOSSIBLE CHILD* by Doris J. Rapp, MD

- Overactivity
- Loudness
- Silliness
- Irritability
- Aggression
- Vulgarity
- Depression
- Hostility
- Fatigue
- Inability to sit still
- Can't concentrate
- Distractibility
- Impulsiveness
- Crawling under furniture
- Hiding in dark corners
- Refusal to be touched
- Abnormal response to directions
- Changes in writing and drawing

Physical Symptoms of Children with Allergies

From *THE IMPOSSIBLE CHILD* by Doris J. Rapp, MD

- Stuffiness
- Clucking throat sounds or throat clearing
- Coughing
- Wheezing
- Itchy or watery eyes
- Swollen eyelids
- Puffy bags below the eyes
- Swollen cracked lips

- Itch skin rashes, especially in arm or leg creases
- Frequent hearing loss following recurrent ear infections
- Sudden ear pain or ringing in the ears
- Recurrent headaches
- Recurrent leg aches or muscle aches
- Wiggling legs, hands or arms
- Recurrent intestinal symptoms such as nausea, bloating, pain, belching, bad breath, rectal gas, diarrhea or constipation.
- Excessive thirst
- Recurrent infections or absenteeism due to "not feeling well"
- Unexplained facial paleness
- Extreme ticklishness

Inconsistent responses to a food can occur. One time there's a reaction and another time there's no reaction. The difference can be due other added ingredients, such as food coloring, or a preservative, or a hidden sugar.

The book *"Why Do I Feel This Way?" - Natural Healing for Optimal Health and Relief from Moods and Depression* is a self-help manual that includes allergy testing, an allergy elimination diet, nutritional planning, and Candida repair. (See Resources)

(You will recall that Candida is due to an overgrowth of yeast in the intestine. Candida's sole source of food is sugar and it causes an intense craving for sugar and dozens of unwanted painful symptoms.)

Additionally, we need to drink **six to eight glasses of water** every day to maintain a healthy nervous system, and reduce stress. Caffeine flushes water from our bodies so it doesn't count as "water". Herbal teas taste good and are good for us, as well.

So you see, our world isn't quite as simple and as healthy as it once was. It takes some education and navigation to know what to eat and what not to eat. Yet, our better grocers are responding to the call for healthier foods. We can now find organic and even farm-fresh foods in many stores.

At first, giving up those non-foods we love may seem like a big challenge, but as we detoxify from these foods, our taste buds change. We come to love healthy natural foods and enjoy the renewed health that comes with eating well.

As to cost, people discover, to their surprise, that they've been spending a lot of money on junk foods. Eating well doesn't have to be expensive. And if it does cost a little more, the extra cost is far less than the medical and drug expenses, along with fewer sick days, that are eliminated, not to mention the long term effects of major health complications.

Our children deserve the best preparation for life they can have. Healthy foods and education can give that to them.

Add in the necessary nutritional food supplements, and you are on the road to optimal health and wellness. It's not rocket science. It's just good sense.

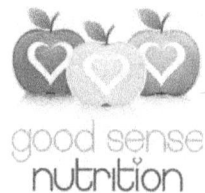

BODY WORK

Periodontal care is a very important step to good health. Inflammation in the gums and tissues of the mouth spreads to the entire body affecting the heart and many organs. Chronic dental inflammation in mid-life can increase heart disease and the risk of Alzheimer's disease.

Sedentary Death Syndrome (SeDS) is a new medical classification. Lack of physical exercise is a major cause of all chronic illness. Physical exercise lowers chronic stress levels. Type II diabetes can almost entirely be prevented by physical exercise.

Stretching isn't about building muscle or losing weight. It's about maintaining a flexible spinal column. The nervous system flows through the spine and when we become stiff and inflexible, the integrity of the spine is compromised, and so is our life. Daily stretching in the morning before other activities can be a life saver, in so many ways. Take a two-minute stretch break every hour that you are sedentary. Notice how your dog and cat stretch after every nap and in between. Just a clue.

Exercise is absolutely necessary for optimal health. Regular exercise can add, not just years to your life, but years of good health while you are living it. Don't like to exercise?

Brisk Non-Stop Walking for 40 minutes, just four days a week, is sufficient. Walking the dog won't cut it. We need to maintain a walk that is fast enough to raise the heart rate and break a little sweat. That's pretty easy, isn't it?

CHRONIC STRESS

Up to 95% of all illness, disease, mental misery, and premature aging is due to chronic stress. To avoid chronic stress, it's important to stay present with what's going on in the moment.

Make your plans for the future, then set them aside. Focus on what's happening right now because "now" is where we live. It's the only place where we can have any effect on life. If we're creating feelings about what happened in the past or about what might happen in the future, we're missing out on what *is* happening right now and now is the only reality. Past and future are really just mental illusions, or mental constructs.

This idea may, or may not, be new to you. It takes practice, for sure. But when we discover how to live in the now, our stress levels decrease and our health improves because we're no longer overwhelmed with mental images, memories, imaginings, thoughts, and feelings.

Conscious breathing is the fastest, easiest, and most effective way to relieve stress. When you're feeling frantic and anxious, practice deep, slow breathing. Expand your rib cage and send the breath deeply into your lungs. Focus only on your breathing. Taking ten deep, slow breaths will relieve anxiety and clear your mind, every time.

a breath of fresh air

INTEGRATIVE MEMORY THERAPY®

See page 53 in the Resources section of this book for information about this powerful resource for discovering the underlying *unconscious* memories that are responsible for many of our moods, behaviors, and physical health issues.

SUMMARY

You now know how food affects moods, bodies, and behaviors. So, what is wellness simplified? Well, here's the bottom line.

WELLNESS SIMPLIFIED

- ELIMINATE SUGARS and ALL WHITE FOODS

- ELIMINATE FAST, JUNK, and PROCESSED FOODS

- TAKE FOOD SUPPLEMENTS REGULARLY

- EAT and ENJOY PROTIEN and HEALTHY FATS

- EAT ORGANIC (if possible) VEGETABLES and FRUITS

- EAT HEALTHY GRAIN PRODUCTS

- DRINK SIX TO EIGHT GLASSES OF WATER DAILY

- STRETCH FREQUENTLY

- EXERCISE FOUR TIMES WEEKLY – Walking is good.

- DO CONSCIOUS DEEP BREATHING OFTEN

In the **PEERS Optimal Health Program** participants found relief and recovery from all of the following disorders using the suggestions I've outlined for you in this book and DVD. I have many written testimonials from grateful men and women whose lives were changed for the better. They didn't find it difficult, because:

It's not a diet. It's not expensive. It's getting one's life back.

Some of the conditions reduced or completely relieved in the PEERS Optimal Health Program were:

ADD/ADHD	Constipation	Memory
Allergies	Depression	Migraines
Anger	Diabetes	Moods
Anxiety	Diarrhea	Motivation
Arthritis	Fibromyalgia	Panic Attacks
Asthma	Gastritis	PMS
Bloating	Hyperactivity	Relationships
Blood Pressure	Insomnia	Skin rashes
Bronchitis	Irritable bowel	Swelling
Candida	Irritability	Ulcers
Cholesterol	Joint pain	Weight gain
Chronic Fatigue	Heart Disease	Weight loss
Concentration	Low Energy	...and more

Participants is the PEERS program were following the same guidelines I've given you in this little book.

One of the participants, Janet Butler, (real name used with permission) wrote, *"We had mountains of guilt that had built up through years of self-doubt and failure, whether it be from weight problems, health problems, or emotional problems. Now we have the tools and resources to be whole. Thank you."*

SUPPORT

Perhaps the information in this book feels challenging to you. If so, that's why **Support** and **Education** are so important. And that's also why I created these Bottom Line Books. I hope you will share this information with others.

I am wishing you a life of health, happiness, and an abundance of all things good. Most sincerely, Dr. Suka

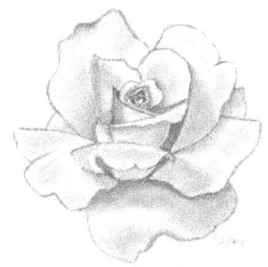

RESOURCES

LABORATORY TESTING

SOME RECOMMENDED TESTS
- DHEA and Cortisol Levels
- Thyroid: TSH, Free T3, Free T4
- Neurotransmitter Levels
- Nutrient Evaluation
- Hormone Levels
- Toxic Metals (Hair and blood analysis)

SUGGESTED LABORTORIES

Direct Health: www.pyroluriatesting.com
A large variety of tests can be ordered directly by the individual on line, through a healthcare provider, or through Dr. Suka. Insurance may cover these tests.

Sanesco Health: www.sanescohealth.com
Sanesco Health offers testing for neurotransmitters and adrenal insufficiency (DHEA and Cortisol). Tests can be ordered through a healthcare provider or through Dr. Suka. Insurance coverage is available.

NeuroScience: www.neurorelief.com
NeuroScience offers neurotransmitter testing. Tests can be ordered through a healthcare provider. Insurance coverage may be available.

Genova Diagnostics: www.gdx.net
Tests can be ordered through a healthcare provider. Insurance coverage may be available.

Life Extension: www.lef.org
Life Extension offers a large variety of tests available to the public without a prescription.

Vitamin D Council: www.vitamindcouncil.com
Inexpensive and accurate Vitamin D testing. No prescription necessary.

TO ORDER HIGH QUALITY SUPPLEMENTS LISTED IN THIS BOOK, CALL ANOVA HEALTH AT 864-408-8320.

Food supplements listed in all of our books can be purchased through Anova Health, also providing WHOLE FOOD supplements. Request a catalog.

Simply call Anova Health and give them the CODE. **Drsuka5** Your order will be shipped the same day, no delays. You will automatically receive a **5% discount and free shipping,** saving you the extra cost of buying supplements of the very best quality. To get these benefits, you must call in your order.

All supplements are of the highest quality available and are suitable for vegetarians. They are free of wheat gluten, soy, milk/dairy, corn, sodium, sugar, starch, artificial coloring, preservatives, and flavoring. I highly recommend the following supplements available through Anova Health.

Amino Acids: All of the amino acids that are listed in my two "how-to" manuals and other books can be ordered through Anova Health. Of course, they can be purchased in many other places, but for the highest quality and purest products, I recommend Anova Health. You may pay a little more, but you will use less and get better results with high quality products.

AvinoCort for managing elevated Cortisol levels caused by chronic stress. Lowering one's cortisol level slows down the aging process and helps to prevent dementia and Alzheimer's. Why use this product? This is a very advanced, stem cell product. Ask the folks at Anova Health for more information if you like. I highly recommend this product for reducing the effects of chronic stress.

Inositol Powder is a normal vitamin B. It is a precursor to GABA, the brain's natural Valium. If you have anxiety, worries, even panic attacks, your inositol level is probably too low. Taking 1000 mg up to four times daily can improve relaxation and reduce anxiety, naturally.

High Potency Hemp Oil with Cannabidiol (CBD): Legal everywhere and has no measurable THC or psycho-active effects. Cannabidiol relieves or cures over 100 symptoms and disorders. Comes as oil and capsules. An excellent balm is also available for topical use. To learn more about the advantages of hemp oil with Cannabidiol versus marijuana with TCH for medicinal support, order the book *Cannabinoids – The Hundredth Monkey Cure* available on our web site. This product, combined with vitamin D3, may be the closest there is to "magic medicine". Recommended for drug and alcohol detoxing and recovery, as well.

CaliQuil - California Poppy 500 mg Capsules Restores Rest. Prevails over pain. Traditional analgesic and sleep aid. This amazing product really works. Take it before bedtime and see the results. (Does not produce opium, physical dependence, or addiction.)

Acute Pain Relief, a King Bio homeopathic cream, gives excellent relief from joint pain.

Call 864-408-8320 to order these and other products from Anova Health. (If you order on-line, you won't get the discount or free shipping.)

Use the code **drsuka5** to order.

OTHER SUGGESTED RESOURCES FOR QUALITY SUPPLEMENTS
Call and request free catalogs. Order by telephone or on-line.

Life Extension: www.lef.org 1-800-678-8989

Bronson Vitamins: www.bronsonvitamins.com 1-800-235-3200

Cayenne Company: www.cayennecompany.com 1-800-229-3663

For highest quality amino acids call: Dr. Suka at 417-380-3254 or 417-894-8501

THREE ALCOHOL RECOVERY PROGRAMS

ARISE **Alcohol Recovery** offers two Do-It-Yourself, at home, recovery programs. These include both a Self-Managed Program and a Managed Program.

ARISE **Alcohol Recovery** also offers an Out-patient Program for individuals who have been through one or more treatment programs, or have made good attempts at recovery through AA, and have relapsed. The program can also serve as an aftercare program for someone coming out of treatment but who is not yet ready to return home.

All programs are based on biochemical restoration of the brain using micronutrient and nutrition therapy, body work, whole life skills, and Integrative Memory Therapy®.

For more information and testimonials, go to:
www.AriseAlcoholRecovery.com

INTEGRATIVE MEMORY THERAPY®

Present day physical, emotional, and mental pain and suffering are the result of unresolved issues from our past. It can be called Post Traumatic Stress. That "past" can be yesterday, or years ago. The unresolved issues may have occurred during our early formative years or in the womb.

Yes, we recorded the feelings, thoughts, and words mother experienced during the time we were a tiny fetus in her womb. We simply recorded these, and all that we saw, heard, and felt during the first seven years of our life. These experiences became our history and our truths because we didn't yet have a conscious mind to discriminate. The stories created beliefs about ourselves and our ability to live in the world, even though the beliefs may have been wrong or harmful.

Sometimes these memories or "stories" may appear to be past life trauma stories that are seeking resolution. It makes no difference whether the stories are fantasy or real. If the stories coming from our own unconscious mind are left unresolved, they create unhealthy survival patterns and suffering in our present lives. These unhealthy survival patterns can show up as addictions, cancer, arthritis, anorexia, depression, PTSD, AD(H)D, for example. In fact, every illness and every disorder is the result of unresolved prior trauma.

Integrative Memory Therapy® gets to the originating source of present day issues, allowing for healing and transformation. Unlike other medical and alternative modalities, this process resolves the root of the problem. Healing in the present takes place because the underlying cause is no longer present.

Integrative Memory Therapy® is not regression, nor is it hypnosis. Clients are fully conscious at all times. The therapist guides clients to resolve their own source traumas. The result is a transformed life in the present. This therapy must be conducted in person. It cannot be conducted via Skype or telephone.

For more information contact Dr. Suka at 417-890-3254 or go to www.IMRIWellness.org. More information and testimonials are available on the web site.

RECOMMENDED BOOKS, DVDs

WORKBOOK   (180 pages)
"Why Do I Feel This Way?"
Natural Relief from Moods and Depression
by Suka Chapel-Horst, RN, PhD, QMHP, CPLT

Moods, cravings, chronic depression, aches, pains and other symptoms are caused by treatable and reversible deficiencies in brain chemistry.

If your brain is low in "feel good" chemicals, you may experience moodiness, sadness, anxiety, overeating, insomnia, irritability, anger, lack of focus and concentration, poor memory, loneliness, decreased sex drive, lack of motivation, racing thoughts, suicidal thoughts, and more.

Find out which "feel good" brain chemicals you may be deficient in. Experience the power of amino acids to restore brain chemistry without medications. Discover the foods and basic food supplements that can restore your life to normal. The guidelines are clear, easy to understand and follow. This book may be all you need to achieve optimal health.

Avoid medication side effects, serious dangers, and addictive qualities. The only way to restore optimal health is by deleting poisonous nonfoods and feeding the brain the natural substances it needs to function normally.

The book includes:
- Ten Written Tests to Uncover the Underlying Cause
- Neurotransmitter Testing
- Amino Acid Formulas
- Nutritional Co-Factor Formulas
- Three Nutritional Programs
- Allergy and Candida Repair
- Seventeen Fun and Effective Stress-Reducing Exercises

WORKBOOK   (179 pages)
How to Quit Drinking for Good and Feel Good
by Suka Chapel-Horst, RN, PhD, QMHP, CPLT

Live at Home

Keep it Private

Continue Normal Activities

Make it Affordable

Much of what we thought we knew about alcoholism and substance abuse is now obsolete. Neuroscience and biochemistry have found the underlying cause of all addictions and thirty-plus years of experience have given us the recovery method that is getting up to 85% recovery rates.

Shame, blame, and guilt be gone. Anger and hurt can change to healing, compassion and forgiveness when the real cause of addictions is understood. Addictions are not caused by a mental illness, nor are they caused by a lack of will power, a character defect, or a moral weakness.

Sobriety is not recovery. "One day at a time" struggling, white knuckling, dry drunk behaviors, depression, insomnia, anxiety, cravings, and other symptoms lead to relapse. With the new understanding of addictions, these, and other symptoms can be relieved and prevented, naturally, without the side effects and addictive qualities of prescription medications.

This book contains ten written tests to determine one's underlying biochemical imbalances, plus individual neurotransmitter tests, and a step-by-step guide for gaining and maintaining lasting recovery without the symptoms that lead to relapse. Normal brain chemistry is restored with the natural building blocks of amino acids, micronutrients and healthy nutrition. This program uses the most successful method of recovery available anywhere. Motivated and determined individuals can recover once and for all.

Written tests included in this book are:
- Alcohol Screening
- Carbohydrate Addiction
- Hypoglycemia
- Hypothyroid
- Candida
- Allergies
- Pyroluria
- High Histamine
- Low Histamine
- Attention Deficit (Hyperactivity) Disorder
- Neurotransmitter Deficiencies

DVD

Depression Cure

Ten Different Sources / Ten Different Approaches   Get Real Results

Your Guide to Finding and Treating the Real Underlying Cause

PowerPoint Presentation by Suka Chapel-Horst, RN, PhD, QMHP, CPLT

Don't waste time using the wrong approach to recovery. "Dr. Suka" pinpoints the different underlying sources of depression which must be treated uniquely and appropriately in order to fully recover without the use of pharmaceuticals. These inter-related causes require different treatment approaches to achieve permanent cure. Don't waste precious time, money, and hopes. Get to the root source from the start and find out how to recover naturally. DVD comes with a resource list.

BOOK (234 pages)
Take a Leap of Faith
Wellness Simplified
by Suka Chapel-Horst, RN, PhD, QMHP, CPLT

If your emotional, mental, or physical health isn't what you wish it to be, you'll find practical suggestions for regaining or maintaining optimal health in this remarkable book. The topics include:

- Halt Premature Aging Now
- Want More Sunshine in Your Life?
- The Cookie Monster - Hypoglycemia
- Five Simple Steps to Optimal Health
- Enjoy Life More
- Your Body Type: Seven Dwarfs and Superman
- Fear versus Love
- Relief from Depression
- Stretching to Wellness
- Bodyguards Got You Covered?
- Bodyguard Banquet
- What are you Hoarding in your Mental House?
- Prevent Dementia and Alzheimer's
- The Hundredth Monkey Cure – Cannabinoids
- Is There a Cure for Alcoholism?
- Color – The Hidden Persuader
- The Ultimate Healing – Integrative Memory and Past Lives Therapy®
- Take a Leap of Faith
- What I know for Sure
- ...and more

In the most delightful and warm way, Dr. Suka "talks" about the topics closest to our minds and hearts.   This book includes transcripts from 24 of her recent Unity.FM international radio shows. You won't want to put this book down.

BOTTOM LINE BOOKS

BOOK
Say Goodbye to Moods and Depression
by Suka Chapel-Horst, RN, PhD, QMHP, CPLT

The only way to restore optimal health is by deleting poisonous nonfoods and feeding the brain the natural substances from which it is made.

Babies are made from food, not Prozac. After birth, why do we switch from the natural building blocks of life to synthetic pills? We can achieve optimal health when we remove the underlying brain chemical imbalances which lead to the symptoms of moods and depression including insomnia, anxiety, panic reactions, irritability, weight gain, aches and pains, and more.

The good news is that targeted micronutrients and healthy nutrition, along with other holistic methods of healthcare, can reduce or eliminate moods and depression, naturally.

BOOK
The Real Cause and Solution for Alcohol Addiction
The NEW Alcoholism Story
by Suka Chapel-Horst, RN, PhD, QMHP, CPLT

Alcohol addiction is caused by an inherited and genetically caused imbalance of brain chemistry. It's not caused by a character defect, a moral shortcoming, or by a lack of will power.

Neuroscience and biochemistry have proven, once and for all, that all addictions are biochemically caused. It's time to give up shame, blame, and guilt for a disorder that is biochemically caused.

When dysfunctional brain chemistry is restored to normal, relapse and dry-drunk symptoms are rare. Learn how imbalanced brain chemistry leads to alcoholism and discover the recovery method that has the highest long-term relapse-free recovery rate.

BOOK
PTSD – Post-Traumatic Stress Disorder
Alternative Resources for Recovery
by Suka Chapel-Horst, RN, PhD, QMHP, CPLT

Medications have long term, harmful side effects, including addiction, and traditional counseling methods are often only partially effective.

There are two underlying causes of PTSD. 1) Biochemical deficiencies, or brain chemistry imbalances, and 2) underlying, UNCONSCIOUS, unresolved trauma which occurred PRIOR to the known trauma-experience that *appears* to be the cause of PTSD. These unconscious memories are called *source trauma.*

Addressing biochemical, nutritional, brain wave state, and bioenergy fields is a necessary component to recovery, including the clearing of destructive cellular memories using the latest science of energy psychology.

Uncovering and resolving hidden source trauma, the underlying cause of PTSD, is accomplished with *Integrative Memory Therapy®.* (See page 39 in this Appendix.)

BOOK
The Gift – A Sound Mind for Life
by Suka Chapel-Horst, RN, PhD, QMHP, CPLT

How to increase mental focus, improve memory, and prevent or delay Alzheimer's. Find out about the effects of stress and how to minimize it in order to prolong health and quality life. The DVD includes biochemical, nutritional, physical, emotional, and mental resources to minimize and delay the effects of aging. This is valuable information for any age.

BOOK
Cannabinoids – The Hundredth Monkey Cure
by Suka Chapel-Horst, RN, PhD, QMHP, CPLT

The human body naturally produces cannabis-like chemicals that keep all body systems in balance. This internal cannabinoid system may be the most important health discovery of recent years. THC, CBN, and CBD from the cannabis sativa plant mimic our internal chemicals and work to improve our overall health. Cannabidiol, or CBD, cures or relieves symptoms of over 100 disorders. ...and it's legal everywhere because it doesn't have the psycho-active ingredient, THC.

Want better natural solutions for your health concerns? This DVD shows how to change brain chemistry and improve your life by using Cannabidiol (CBD), amino acids, neuronutrients, nutrition, exercise, and chronic stress reducers. Say goodbye to anxiety, stress, depression, insomnia, pain, physical disorders, and much more.

BOOK
Trick or Treat – What Your Doctor isn't Telling You about Mood Altering Medications
by Suka Chapel-Horst, RN, PhD, QMHP, CPLT

Is your doctor treating you or tricking you? If you are considering taking mood altering medications, are already on them, or want to get off them, you need to know what these medications are really doing to brain chemistry. Be informed in order to make wise decisions. Your emotional and mental life is at stake.

These books and DVDs can be ordered through:
www.IMRIWellness.org
www.AriseAlcoholRecovery.com
Or by calling: 417-380-3254